GREENS

DON'T GROW IN CANS

WRITTEN & ILLUSTRATED BY:
AMANDA M. MACK

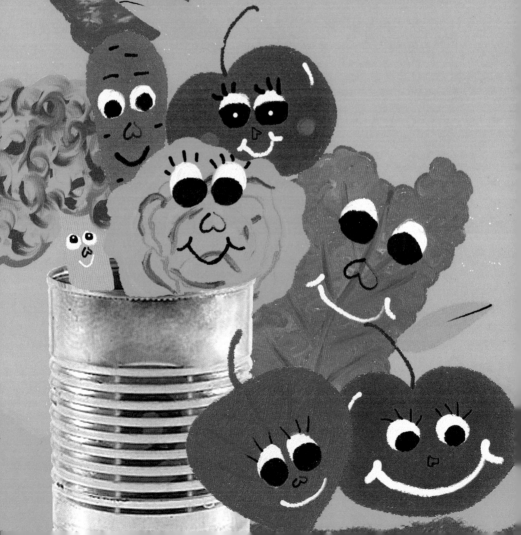

Greens Don't Grow In Cans
© 2014 Amanda M. Mack

ISBN-13: 978-1511825658
ISBN-10: 1511825650

Library of Congress Control Number: 2015906499
CreateSpace Independent Publishing Platform,
North Charleston, SC

Printed in the United States

This book is dedicated to my children; Jarrod & Autumn Mack. With all of my heart, I love you! Continue to love, support and nurture one another as you grow into beautiful beings. May your smiles reflect happiness that touches others. Thanks to my rock, my husband as well as my family and friends! I could not have done this without you.

APPLES GROW ON TREES
WAY UP HIGH.

WHEN THEY ARE RIPE
ENOUGH THEY FALL FROM
THE SKY.

SWEET AND JUICY WHEN
YOU BITE, BUT THERE IS
MORE TO SAY.

THEY ARE SO YUMMY
FULL OF VITAMIN A!

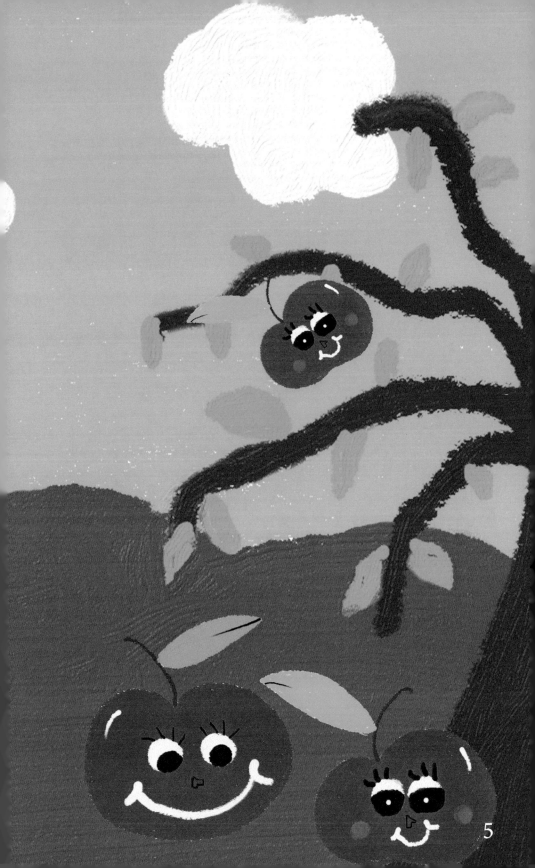

CARROTS GROW UNDERGROUND NOT INSIDE A CAN.

THEIR SPROUTS PUSH THROUGH THE SOIL.

PULL THEM WITH YOUR HANDS!

TASTE THEM! THEY ARE BRIGHT AND CRUNCHY. YOU WILL BE SURPRISED,

TO KNOW THAT EATING THEM HELPS YOUR EYES.

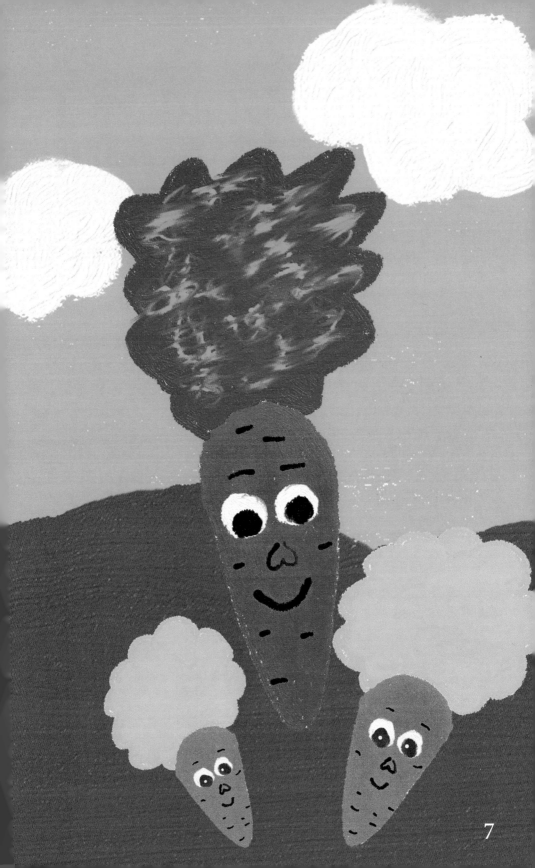

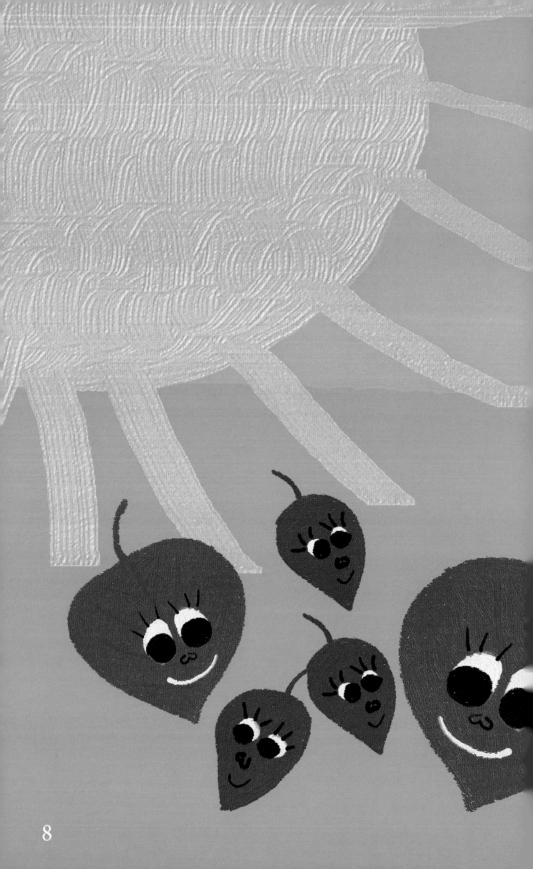

8

SPINACH GROWS IN THE SOIL AND LOOKS LIKE A LEAF.

BITE SOME LIKE A CATERPILLAR WITH YOUR TEETH!

FULL OF VITAMIN K AND B, STEAM THEM IN A PAN.

AND NEVER FORGET, GREENS DON'T GROW IN CANS!

KALE ARE PART OF THE
BRASSICA BUNCH.

GROWN FROM THE
GROUND AND EATEN UP
FOR LUNCH,

OR DINNER TIME,
BREAKFAST TIME,

A SMOOTHIE IS THE WAY,
TO DRINK UP YOUR
VITAMINS A, C AND K!

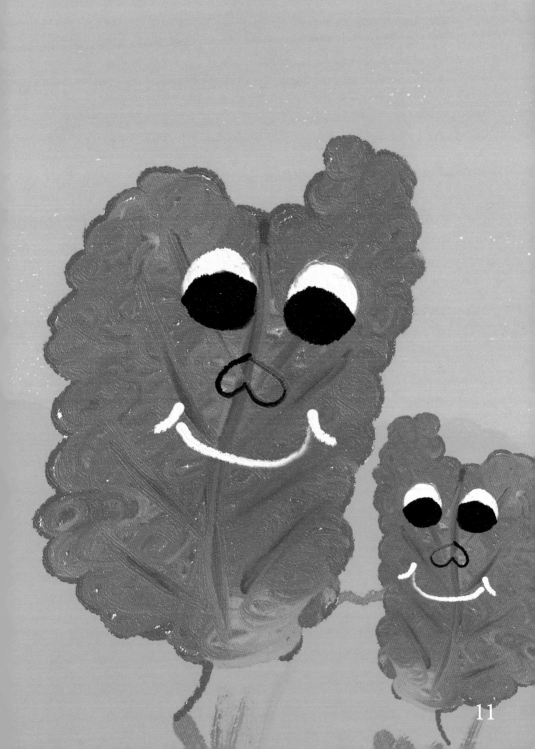

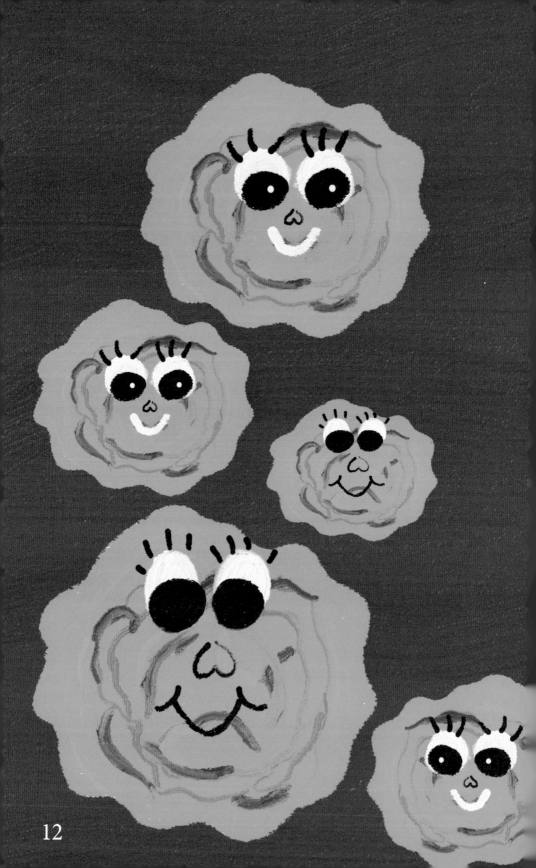

CABBAGE GROWS IN THE
SOIL SOME PURPLE AND
SOME GREEN.

WITH LOTS OF LAYERS
SCRUB IT GOOD TO MAKE
SURE IT IS CLEAN.

PEEL OFF ONE LEAF AND
UP COMES ANOTHER,

EAT IT UP FOR B6,
JUST GET HELP FROM
MOTHER!

BROCCOLI IS A
VEGETABLE MY FAVORITE
ONE SO FAR.

STEAM IT OR DIP IT, AND
EAT IT UP RAW!

HOWEVER YOU SHOULD
CHOOSE,
FRESHER IS THE KEY

TO ALWAYS GET THE MOST
VITAMIN C

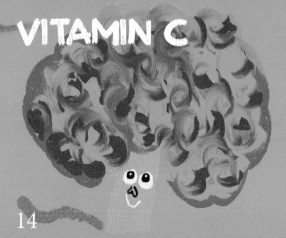

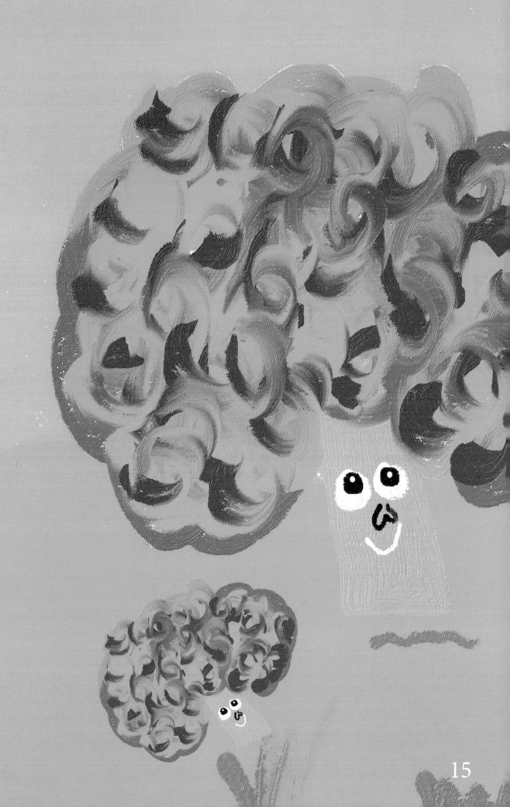

FRESH FRUITS AND
VEGGIES ARE GOOD FOR
YOU!

THEY KEEP YOU STRONG
AND HEALTHY TOO.

16

FROM FARM TO TABLE, I HOPE YOU UNDERSTAND.

THE HEALTHIEST AND FRESHEST GREENS DON'T GROW IN CANS!

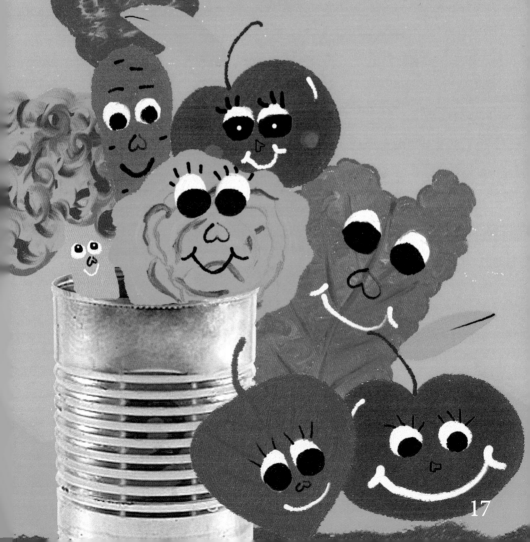

GREENS GROW IN SOIL,
ON VINES AND IN
BUNCHES

SO GOOD THAT INSECTS
AND ANIMAL MUNCHES.

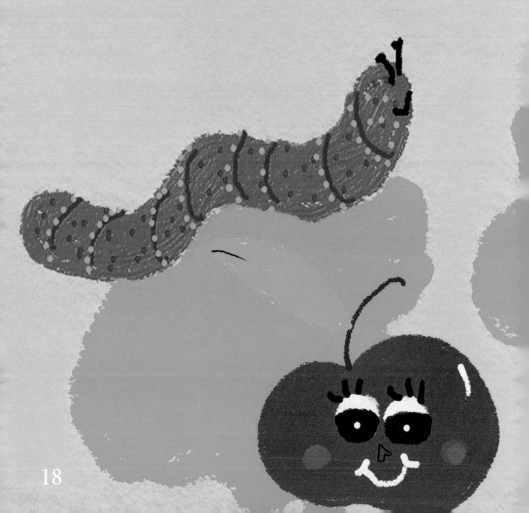

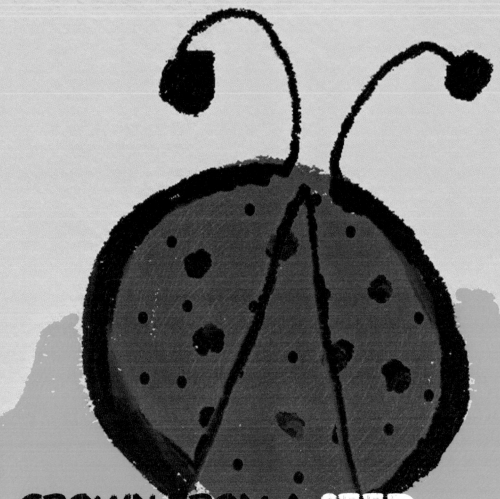

GROWN FROM A **SEED**,
SOME PLANTED BY
HAND.

ITS NOT A SECRET
GREENS DON'T GROW IN
CANS!

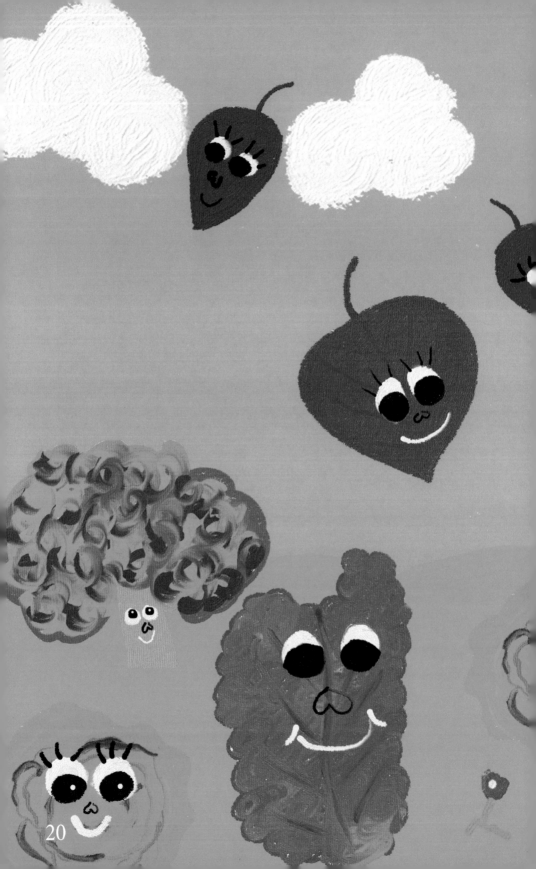

20

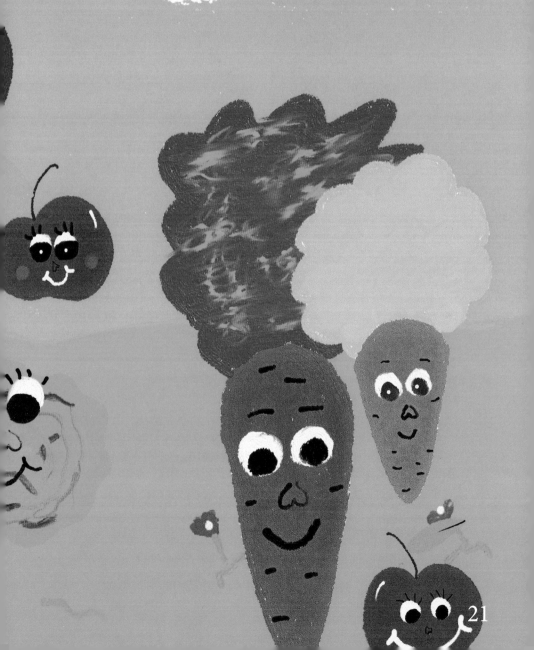

CAN YOU NAME THEM ALL?
GIVE IT A TRY!

Dear Parents,

Can goods also known as non-perishable items, offer extensive preservation of common fruits and vegetables. Many food banks and drives utilize nonperishable items, to serve people with access to limited or no food sources. Non-perishable items, though convenient for many, should not replace the recommended daily value of fresh fruits and vegetables.

Because **Greens Don't Grow In Cans**, as parents we must educate our children on the birthplace of fresh foods. Teach them how these foods sustain and promote growth within their bodies and most importantly, EAT fresh foods with them.

When possible, shop at local farms and farmers markets for access to the freshest produce. Fruits and vegetables purchased locally, are generally 'farm to table' within three days. Imported produce purchased at your local supermarket, could be picked more than eight days before you get it home.

I hope that **Greens Don't Grow In Cans** is a great start to a healthy lifestyle for you and your family! Let's Grow Together!

Amanda M. Mack

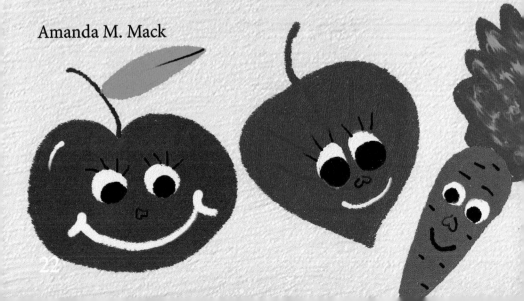

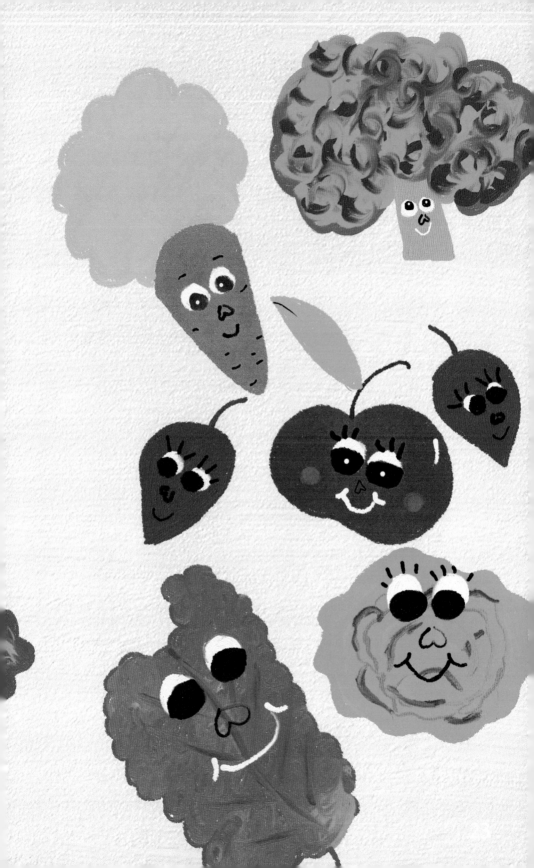

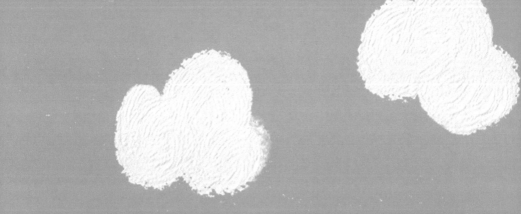

Food is intended to nourish, preserve and protect your body. In its natural state, fresh fruits and vegetables provide you with an enormous amount of nutritional benefits.

Greens Don't Grow In Cans, teaches the origin and nutritional value of fresh fruits and vegetables in an artistic and exciting way! Let's Grow Together!

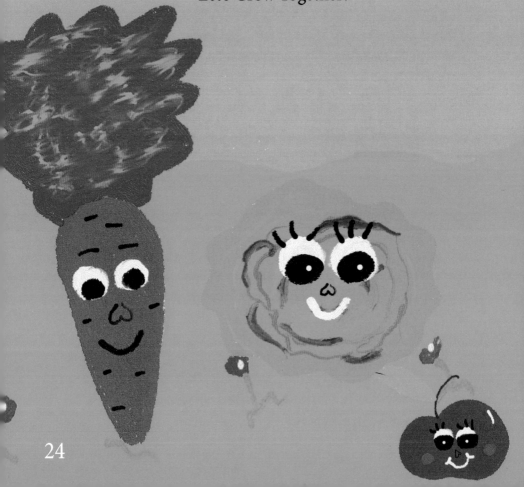

Made in the USA
Charleston, SC
30 April 2015